Table of Contents

Introduction 3

Bone Cancer 4

Primary Bone Cancer 6

Secondary Bone Cancer 7

Bone Cancer Symptoms 8

Bone Cancer Diagnosis 9

Bone Cancer Treatment 10

Prevention 12

When to see a doctor 13

Risk factors 13

Bone Tumor 14

Benign Bone Tumors 18

Recipes 19

PHO-FLAVORED PRESSURE COOKER BONE BROTH 19

Easy Potato Soup 22

Cancer Fighting Soup 23

How to Make Beef Broth 27

How to Make Bone Broth 30

Slow Cooker Chicken Stock 34

Beef Bone Broth Recipe 35

Anti-Cancer Green Smoothie Recipe 37

Mac and Cheese 39

Apple Pie Smoothie 41

Baked Eggs with Tomatoes and Mozzarella 41

Baked French Toast 43

Banana Pancakes 45

Barley Risotto 47

Black Beans, Corn, and Quinoa Salad 49

Breakfast Egg Cups 51

Black Beans, Corn, and Quinoa Salad 52

Brown Rice Stir Fry 54

Buffalo Cauliflower Bites 56

Butternut Squash and Apple Soup 58

Cantaloupe and Mint Granita 60

Butternut Squash and Apple Soup 62

Buffalo Cauliflower Bites 64

Brown Rice Stir Fry 66

Buffalo Cauliflower Bites 68

Butternut Squash and Apple Soup 69

Cantaloupe and Mint Granita 72

Rainbow Grain Bowl with Cashew Tahini Sauce 73

Herbed Avocado Egg Salad 76

Lentil Soup 78

Mango Lassi 80

Quinoa Salad with Feta 81

Herbed Avocado Egg Salad 83

Introduction

Bone cancer can begin in any bone in the body, but it most commonly affects the pelvis or the long bones in the arms and legs. Bone cancer is rare, making up less than 1 percent of all cancers. In fact, noncancerous bone tumors are much more common than cancerous ones. The term "bone cancer" doesn't include cancers that begin elsewhere in the body and spread (metastasize) to the bone. Instead, those cancers are named for where they began, such as breast cancer that has metastasized to the bone. Some types of bone cancer occur primarily in children, while others affect mostly adults. Surgical removal is the most common treatment, but chemotherapy and radiation therapy also may be utilized. The decision to use surgery, chemotherapy or radiation therapy is based on the type of bone cancer being treated. Bone cancer, disease characterized by uncontrolled growth of cells of the bone. Primary bone cancer—that is, cancer that arises directly in the bone—is relatively rare. In the United States, for example, only about 3,600 new cases of primary bone cancer are diagnosed each year. Most cancer that involves the bone is cancer that has spread (metastasized) from other tissues in the body through the blood or lymphatic systems. Different types of bone tissue give rise to different types of primary bone cancer. Osteosarcoma develops from cells that form the bone, and Ewing tumour of the bone (Ewing sarcoma) develops from immature nerve tissue within the bone. Both types most commonly affect males between 10 and 20 years of age. Chondrosarcoma, which forms in cartilage tissue, principally affects persons over age 50. More than one-half of the cases of primary bone cancer, even once-deadly types, can now be treated successfully.

Bone Cancer

Bone cancer is when unusual cells grow out of control in your bone. It destroys normal bone tissue. It may start in your bone or spread there from other parts of your body (called metastasis).

Bone cancer is rare. Most bone tumors are benign, which means they aren't cancer and don't spread to other areas of your body. But they may still weaken your bones and lead to broken bones or other problems. There are a few common types of benign bone tumors:

• Osteochondroma is the most common. It often happens in people under age 20.

• Giant cell tumor is usually in your leg. In rare cases, these can also be cancerous.

• Osteoid osteoma often happens in long bones, usually in your early 20s.

• Osteoblastoma is a rare tumor that grows in your spine and long bones, mostly in young adults.

• Enchondroma usually appears in bones of your hands and feet. It often has no symptoms. It's the most common type of hand tumor.

Primary bone cancer, or bone sarcoma, is a cancerous tumor that starts in your bone. Experts aren't sure what causes it, but your genes may play a role. Some of the most common types of primary bone cancer are:

• Osteosarcoma often forms around your knee and upper arm. Teens and young adults are most likely to get it, but another form is common in adults who have Paget's disease of bone.

• Ewing's sarcoma usually happens in people between the ages of 5 and 20. Your ribs, pelvis, leg, and upper arm are the most common sites. It can also start in the soft tissue around your bones.

• Chondrosarcoma happens most often in people between ages 40 and 70. Your hip, pelvis, leg, arm, and shoulder are common sites of this cancer, which begins in cartilage cells.

• Although it happens in your bones, multiple myeloma is not a primary bone cancer. It's a cancer of your marrow, the soft tissue inside bones.

Secondary Bone Cancer

Cancer in your bones usually started elsewhere in your body. For example, if lung cancer has spread to your bones, that's secondary bone cancer. Any cancer that moves from one part of your body to another is called metastatic cancer.

Cancers that commonly spread to bone include:

• Breast cancer

• Prostate cancer

• Lung cancer

• Bone Cancer Risk Factors

Things that might make you more likely to get bone cancer include:

Cancer treatment. Bone tumors happen more often in people who've had radiation, stem cell transplants, or certain chemotherapy drugs for other cancers.

Inherited conditions. Diseases passed down through your genes, such as Li-Fraumeni syndrome and an eye cancer called retinoblastoma, can make you more likely to get bone cancer.

Bone Cancer Symptoms

You may not notice symptoms of a bone tumor, whether it's cancer or not. Your doctor might find it when they look at an X-ray of another problem, such as a sprain. But symptoms can include pain that:

• Is in the area of the tumor

• Is dull or achy

• Gets worse with activity

• Wakes you at night

• An injury won't cause a bone tumor.

Other symptoms related to bone tumors include:

• Fevers

• Night sweats

• Swelling around a bone

• Limping

• Fatigue

• Weight loss

Bone Cancer Diagnosis

Your doctor will ask about your symptoms and medical history and do a physical exam. They'll look at pictures of your bones through imaging tests such as:

• X-rays. These show tumors and how big they are.

• CT scans. A computer uses X-rays to make more detailed pictures.

• MRI scans. These use a strong magnet to show inside your body.

• PET scans. A technician injects radioactive glucose (sugar) into your vein. A scanner then spots cancer cells, which use more glucose than regular cells.

• Bone scans. A technician injects a different radioactive material into your vein. It collects in your bones, where a scanner can see it.

Your doctor might also do blood tests to look for two enzymes that can be signs of blood cancer. A procedure called a biopsy can confirm a diagnosis. Your doctor takes a sample of the tumor with a needle or through a cut in your skin. A trained technician looks at the tissue or cells under a microscope. They can tell if your tumor is benign or a primary or secondary cancer. They can also get an idea of how fast it's growing.

Bone Cancer Treatment

If you have a benign tumor, your doctor will treat it with medication or might just watch it for changes. They may take out benign tumors that are more likely to spread or become cancer. In some cases, tumors come back, even after treatment.

Cancerous tumors need stronger treatment and care from a number of specialists. Your treatment will depend on several things including how far it's spread, which experts use to determine its stage. Cancer cells that are only in the bone tumor and the surrounding area are at a "localized" stage. Those that spread to or from other areas of your body are more serious and harder to treat.

Common treatments for bone cancer include:

• Limb salvage surgery. Your doctor removes the part of the bone with cancer but not nearby muscles, tendons, or other tissues. They put a metallic implant in place of the bone.

• Amputation. If a tumor is large or reaches your nerves and blood vessels, your doctor might remove the limb. You may get a prosthetic limb afterward.

• Radiation therapy. This kills cancer cells and shrinks tumors with strong X-rays. Doctors often use it along with surgery.

• Chemotherapy. This kills tumor cells with cancer drugs. Your doctor might use it before surgery, after surgery, or for metastatic cancer.

• Targeted therapy. This drug treatment targets certain genetic, protein, or other changes in or around cancer cells.

Prevention

Prevention of bone cancer will require a better understanding of its causes than is currently available. If a patient has a known risk factor for bone cancer, such as Paget disease, careful screening may help detect and treat the cancer in its early stages, thereby improving the chances for survival.

Symptoms

Signs and symptoms of bone cancer include:

- Bone pain

- Swelling and tenderness near the affected area

- Weakened bone, leading to fracture

- Fatigue

- Unintended weight loss

When to see a doctor

Make an appointment with your doctor if you or your child develops bone pain that:

- Comes and goes

- Becomes worse at night

- Isn't helped by over-the-counter pain relievers

Risk factors

It's not clear what causes bone cancer, but doctors have found certain factors are associated with an increased risk, including:

• Inherited genetic syndromes. Certain rare genetic syndromes passed through families increase the risk of bone cancer, including Li-Fraumeni syndrome and hereditary retinoblastoma.

• Paget's disease of bone. Most commonly occurring in older adults, Paget's disease of bone can increase the risk of bone cancer developing later.

• Radiation therapy for cancer. Exposure to large doses of radiation, such as those given during radiation therapy for cancer, increases the risk of bone cancer in the future.

Bone Tumor

Bone tumors develop when cells within a bone divide uncontrollably, forming a lump or mass of abnormal tissue. Most bone tumors are benign (not cancerous). Benign tumors are usually not life-threatening and, in most cases, will not spread to other parts of the body. Depending upon the type of tumor, treatment options are wide-ranging — from simple observation to surgery to remove the tumor. Some bone tumors are malignant (cancerous). Malignant bone tumors can metastasize — or cause cancer cells to spread throughout the body. In almost all cases, treatment for malignant tumors involves a combination of chemotherapy, radiation, and surgery.

Bone tumors can affect any bone in the body and develop in any part of the bone — from the surface to the center of the bone, called the bone marrow. A growing bone tumor — even a benign tumor — destroys healthy tissue and weakens bone, making it more vulnerable to fracture.

When a bone tumor is cancerous, it is either a primary bone cancer or a secondary bone cancer.

A primary bone cancer actually begins in bone

A secondary bone cancer begins somewhere else in the body and then metastasizes or spreads to bone. Secondary bone cancer is also called metastatic bone disease.

Types of cancer that begin elsewhere and commonly spread to bone include:

• Breast

• Lung

• Thyroid

• Renal (kidney)

• Prostate

• Primary Bone Cancer

The four most common types of primary bone cancer are:

Multiple myeloma. Multiple myeloma is the most common primary bone cancer. It is a malignant tumor of bone marrow — the soft tissue in the center of many bones that produces blood cells. Any bone can be affected by this cancer.

Multiple myeloma affects approximately seven people per 100,000 each year. According to the National Cancer Institute, more than

130,000 people are living with the disease each year. Most cases are seen in patients between the ages of 50 and 70. Multiple myeloma is typically treated with chemotherapy, radiation therapy and, occasionally, surgery.

Osteosarcoma. Osteosarcoma is the second most common primary bone cancer. It occurs in two to five people per million each year, with most cases in teenagers and children. Most tumors develop around the knee in either the femur (thighbone) or tibia (shinbone). Other common locations include the hip and shoulder. Osteosarcoma is typically treated with chemotherapy and surgery.

Ewing's sarcoma. Ewing's sarcoma usually occurs in patients between the ages of 5 and 20. The most common locations affected are the upper and lower leg, pelvis, upper arm, and ribs. Ewing's sarcoma is typically treated with chemotherapy and either surgery or radiation therapy.

Chondrosarcoma. Chondrosarcoma is a malignant tumor composed of cartilage-producing cells. It is most often seen in patients between the ages of 40 and 70. Most cases occur around the hip, pelvis, or shoulder area. In most cases, surgery is the only treatment used for chondrosarcoma.

Benign Bone Tumors

There are many types of benign bone tumors, as well as some diseases and conditions that resemble bone tumors. Although these conditions are not truly bone tumors, in many cases they require the same treatment.

Some common types of benign bone tumors — and conditions that are commonly grouped with tumors — include:

• Nonossifying fibroma

• Unicameral (simple) bone cyst

• Osteochondroma

- Giant cell tumor

- Enchondroma

- Fibrous dysplasia

- Chondroblastoma

- Aneurysmal bone cyst

- Osteoid osteoma

Recipes

PHO-FLAVORED PRESSURE COOKER BONE BROTH

INGREDIENTS

- 1–2 yellow/sweet onions

- 1 piece ginger

- 1/2 – 1 tsp coconut oil

- 2 Tbsp fish sauce

- 1–2 Tbsp salt

- 1 – 1 1/2 lbs bones – You can use beef, ox tail, or turkey necks, or a combination. Combination is great, and ox tail is my favorite for flavor, but just use whatever you have in your freezer. I use whatever I can fit in the IP. 1-1.5 lbs is probably good.

- Spices – I don't usually measure …so I'm guessing the amounts.

- maybe 5 stars, or 1 tsp star anise

- about 1 tsp cloves

- 1 tsp black peppercorn – just use a tsp for everything…

- 1 cinnamon stick

- 1 tsp cardamom pods

- 1 tsp fennel seeds

- 1 tsp coriander seeds

INSTRUCTIONS

- Chop 1 or 2 onions in half.

• Chop 1 piece of ginger in half lengthwise, so that the good stuff is showing.

• Broil in oven onions and ginger until charred – maybe 10 min or so. Have your fan on so everytime you check your smoke detector doesn't go off.

• While all this is going on, get out your spices. In a non-stick pan, combine all that on low heat until they are fragrant – 3-4 min. Always stir – burnt spices will wreck everything.

• Turn Instant Pot onto SAUTE and wait for it to heat up. Add some coconut oil and brown your bones. You will brown these bones on all sides [turn as needed].

• As you are doing this, boil water in kettle – this makes the process faster.

• Once your bones are browned, turn IP off. Add boiled water, onions and ginger, spices and fish sauce, and salt to taste – probably 1-2 Tbsp.

• Fill remainder of Instant Pot with boiled water to max line (or cold water, it'll just take longer).

• [Turn InstantPot to] manual setting for 75 min and use a slow pressure release.

• Strain and put into jars. I like to freeze mine and thaw them as needed.

Easy Potato Soup

This potato soup is simple to make. The flavor and texture can help when you have taste changes or an upset stomach but can also be enjoyed when you're feeling great. Bone broth is as mild as chicken or vegetable broth but with more protein, for those days when you need a boost.

Ingredients

• 1 baking potato

• 2 cups bone broth

Instructions

• Preheat oven to 400 degrees. Bake potato for 30 minutes, or until flesh gives slightly when squeezed. Let the potato cool, then remove skin.

• Bring broth to a boil.

• Carefully combine the potato and bone broth in a blender and puree until smooth.

• Serve warm.

Cancer Fighting Soup

This hearty soup brings a healthy and tasty dose of vegetables to the table to boost the immune system. Make ahead and freeze for later using our freezing instructions.

Ingredients

• 1–2 tablespoons olive oil

• 1 onion, diced

• 2–3 celery stalks, sliced

• 2 cups carrots, diced

• 3 garlic cloves

• Salt and pepper, to taste

• 1/4–1/2 teaspoon red pepper flakes (use less if you don't like heat)

• 1 teaspoon dried Italian seasoning

• 12 cups (or three 32-ounce cartons) of chicken or vegetable broth

• 1 28–ounce can of crushed tomatoes (look for BPA-free cans)

• 2 tablespoons tomato paste

• 1 can black beans, drained and rinsed

• 1/2 cup lentils (any kind will work; rinse first)

• 2 bay leaves

• 1 zucchini, diced

- 1 cup mushrooms, diced

- 1 cup cauliflower, chopped finely

- 1 cup broccoli, chopped finely

- 2–3 cups spinach, chopped

- 1–2 cups frozen green peas

Before You Begin! If you make this, please leave a review and rating letting us know how you liked this recipe! This helps our business thrive & continue providing free recipes.

Instructions

Make It Now:

- Heat 1-2 tablespoons olive oil in a large stock pot over medium-high heat.

- Saute the onions, carrots, and celery for about 4-5 minutes, until tender. Add in the garlic and stir for 1 more minute. Season with salt, pepper, red pepper flakes (to your preferred heat level), and Italian seasoning.

• Stir in the chicken or vegetable broth, crushed tomatoes, tomato paste, black beans, lentils, and bay leaves. Bring to a boil and reduce to a simmer (slight bubbling), stirring occasionally. Season again lightly with salt and pepper. Let simmer for about 10-15 minutes.

• Stir in the zucchini, mushrooms, cauliflower, and broccoli and simmer another 5-10 minutes.

• Stir in the spinach and frozen peas and turn off the heat (or turn to low), so they don't overcook. Remove bay leaves. Taste and adjust seasonings. (Freezing instructions begin here.)

• If you like, serve with freshly shredded Parmesan cheese and/or whole grain crackers or crusty bread.

• Freeze For Later: Follow steps 1-5. Let the soup cool completely. Suggestion: divide soup into some shallow pans to put in the refrigerator to cool it more quickly. Divide soup into gallon-sized freezer bags or containers, squeeze out excess air, seal, and freeze.

• Prepare From Frozen: Thaw using one of these safe thawing methods. Then reheat gently over low heat on the stove or in a crock pot. Another option is to put the frozen soup block over low to medium-low heat on the stove top or in a crock pot. Add about 1-2 cups of water or broth over the top. Gently warm over low to medium-low heat, stirring occasionally. Follow step 6 for serving.

How to Make Beef Broth

Ingredients

• 1.5 lbs. beef bones (grass-fed), exposed marrow bones or joints preferred (use Home Grown Cow to find beef bones in your area)

• 2 Tbl raw apple cider vinegar, optional (not ideal or necessary for those with FODMAP or fructose sensitivities)

• Filtered water

• 1 Tbl + 2 tsp unrefined sea salt, (adjust according to pot size and to taste)

Instructions

• Add bones to crock-pot.

• Fill with filtered water.

• Add apple cider vinegar and sea salt.

• Once the water is simmering or very hot, cook for 2-3 hours.

• Harvest all fat, or fatty broth, for a healing tonic.

• Add new water, salt, and apple cider vinegar and simmer on low at least 24 hours and up to 72 hours.

• Strain and use.

Carrot Ginger Soup

Ingredients

• 2 tbsp avocado oil

- 1 onion large, diced

- 5 cloves garlic

- 3 tbsp ginger grated

- 4 lbs carrot diced; about 7-8 cups

- 2 apple diced

- 3 cups chicken broth or bone broth, veggie broth; low sodium

- 1/2 cup water

- salt to taste; optional

Instructions

- In a large pot or dutch oven, heat avocado oil over medium heat. Add onion and sauté until translucent, about 5 minutes. Add garlic and ginger and cook for another minute, until fragrant.

- Add carrots, apple, broth, water, and a pinch of salt. Cover and simmer over medium low heat for 20 minutes until carrots are soft.

• Omit the salt for a low sodium version.

• The final step is to blend the soup. This can be done with an immersion blender or in batches using a traditional blender.

• Serve and enjoy!

How to Make Bone Broth

Bone broth is one of those recipes that's going to be a little different every time, and that's just fine. Use whatever bones you have on hand (or get from your butcher), but I strongly recommend you always start with bones from pastured, humanely and sustainably raised animals.

For Molly, I didn't add any vegetables or seasonings, other than bay leaves and vinegar, since we want to keep it as simple as possible for her right now. But for you, I'd suggest adding vegetables, herbs, and spices - a few options are noted in the recipe below.

This recipe can be made on the stove or in a slow-cooker -- but don't try to speed the process with a pressure cooker. The vinegar helps leach out additional nutrients from the bones, and the bay leaves, according to Dr. Palmquist, are "antibacterial and anti-inflammatory, and drain the lymphatic system."

Prep Time 5 minutes

Cook Time 6 hours

Total Time 6 hours 5 minutes

Yield 4 quarts

Ingredients

The Basics

- 2 to 3 pounds bones

- 2 bay leaves

- 1/4 cup apple cider vinegar

- 4 to 6 quarts filtered water

- Veggies

- 2 carrots

- 2 celery stalks

- spring of rosemary and/or thyme

For Humans Only

- 1 onion chopped in large chunks

- 1/2 teaspoon whole peppercorns

- salt to taste (add after cooking)

Instructions

- In the largest pot you own (or in your slow-cooker), add the bones, bay leaves, and vinegar. Fill with water. If making this for people and not for pets, add the onion and peppercorns.

- Bring to a boil, and then skim off any foam that comes to the surface. Turn heat to the lowest possible setting on your stove or slow-cooker, and cover.

• Let simmer for at least 6 hours and up to 72 hours. The larger the bones, the longer you'll want to go. If you're losing a lot of water to evaporation, it's okay to top off with a little extra boiling water.

• If making this for people, add salt to taste, being careful not to burn your tongue

• Allow to cool, and then skim the fat off the top and discard. Strain and pour into jars to store. If storing in the fridge, use within a few days, or store in the freezer for several months.

Recipe Notes

For determining quantity, you'll need to let experience and personal preference be your guide. As a general starting point, figure about two pounds of bones per gallon of water.

Two tips for storing in the freezer: First, you can freeze some in ice-cube trays and then you'll have some small amounts ready-to-go when you need them. Second, if it's at room temperature, you can pour into a zip-top bag and freeze flat in the bag -- just be sure the bag is sealed very well!

Slow Cooker Chicken Stock

Ingredients

• ½ pound chicken bones (see Chef Tips)

• 2 cups onions, chopped

• 1 cup carrots, chopped

• 1 cup celery, chopped

• 2 bay leaves

• 4 sprigs thyme

• 1 splash vinegar, optional (for brightening flavor)

Directions

- In a 3- quart crock pot, add chicken bones, onions, carrots, celery, bay leaves, and thyme. Pour cold water over bones and vegetables to cover, about 8 cups. Cover with the lid and turn on high.

- Cook stock for 8 to 12 hours, skimming fat and foam off top.

- Once cooked and flavorful, strain bones and vegetables from liquid. Chill and store in an airtight container in refrigerator for up to one week or freeze for future use.

Beef Bone Broth Recipe

INGREDIENTS

- 4 pounds beef bones with marrow

- 4 carrots, chopped

- 4 celery stalks, chopped

- 2 medium onions, peel on, sliced in half lengthwise and quartered

- 4 garlic cloves, peel on and smashed

- 1 teaspoon sea salt

- 1 teaspoon whole peppercorns

- 2 bay leaves

- 3 sprigs fresh thyme

- 6 sprigs parsley

- ¼ cup apple cider vinegar

- 20 cups cold water

INSTRUCTIONS

- Place all ingredients in a 10 quart capacity slow cooker or large stock pot on the stove.

- Add in water.

- Turn on the slow cooker and prepare to cook for at least 36 hours, so that might mean 3 cycles on the standard slow cooker that has a maximum 12-hour setting (unless you can set your slow cooker

for 36 hours).

• If cooking on a stovetop, bring the large pot to a boil over high

heat; reduce and simmer gently.

• In slow cooker or pot, skim the fat that rises to the surface

occasionally.

• Simmer for 36 to 48 hours.

• Remove from heat and allow to cool slightly.

• Discard solids and strain remainder in a bowl through a colander.

Let stock cool to room temperature, cover and chill.

• Refrigerate and use within a week. Or freeze for up to 3 months.

Anti-Cancer Green Smoothie Recipe

This Anti-Cancer Green Smoothie recipe is full of health-promoting

ingredients, including leafy greens and broccoli florets. This vegan and dairy-free blended drink can be served as a meal replacement or as a snack. Easy to make and delicious, too.

Ingredients

- 1/4 cup hemp seeds

- 2 cups carrot juice

- 1 cup water

- 1 ripe banana, frozen

- 1 cup frozen strawberries

- 1 cup frozen broccoli florets

- 2 cups fresh or lightly steamed baby kale or baby spinach

- 5 fresh mint leaves

- 2 tablespoons cocoa powder

- 1/2 lime or lemon, juiced

Instructions

• Combine the hemp seeds, carrot juice, and water in the base of a high-speed blender like a Vitamix or Blendtec.

• Next, add the frozen banana, frozen strawberries, frozen broccoli florets, greens, mint, cocoa powder, and lemon or lime juice.

• Place the lid on the blender and blend until smooth, about 45 seconds.

• Serve immediately.

Mac and Cheese

Ingredients

• 1 stick unsalted butter

• 5½ cups milk

• ½ cup unbleached white flour

• 1½ Tbsps. salt

• ¼ tsp. freshly ground black pepper

• 3 cups freshly grated white sharp Cheddar cheese 12 oz.

• 1½ cups freshly grated gruyere 6 oz.

• 2 lbs. elbow macaroni

Instructions

• Fill a large pot with water and bring to a boil. Cook macaroni according to box directions. Drain in a colander and rinse with cold water.

• Heat milk in a medium saucepan over medium heat. In the pasta pot, melt butter over medium heat. When butter bubbles, add flour. Whisk for one minute.

• While whisking, slowly pour in hot milk, whisking constantly until mixture bubbles and thickens.

• Remove from heat. Mix in both cheeses, salt and pepper. Add in reserved macaroni and stir until mixed.

Ingredients

- ½ cup soy, almond, or rice milk

- ½ cup sweetened applesauce

- ½ ripe medium banana

- ¼ teaspoon vanilla extract

- ¼ teaspoon cinnamon

- ½ cup ice cubes (optional)

- 1 scoop whey protein powder (optional)

Instructions

- Combine all ingredients in blender. Pulse until smooth.

Baked Eggs with Tomatoes and Mozzarella

Ingredients

- 2 tablespoons olive oil

- ½ small yellow onion, chopped

- 2 cloves garlic, minced

- 28-ounce can crushed tomatoes

- Salt and pepper

- 4 ounces fresh mozzarella, cut into 1/2-inch pieces

- ¼ cup fresh oregano leaves, coarsely chopped

- 8 eggs

- 4 slices multigrain toast (optional)

Instructions

- Thoroughly rinse fresh produce under warm running water for 20 seconds. Scrub to remove excess dirt.

- Preheat oven to 350 degrees.

- In a saucepan over medium-high heat, warm olive oil. Add onion and cook until translucent, about 5 minutes. Add garlic and cook until fragrant. Stir in tomatoes with juices, season with salt and pepper to taste, and bring to a boil. Reduce heat to low and simmer until nicely thickened, about 15 minutes. Season with more salt and pepper to taste.

• Place four medium ramekins on a baking sheet. Divide tomato sauce evenly between ramekins. Top with mozzarella and oregano. Break 2 eggs into each ramekin, on top of the tomato sauce and cheese, and season with salt and pepper.

• Bake until egg whites are opaque and yolks register as 160 degrees or higher using an instant-read thermometer (set but still slightly runny in the middle), about 15 minutes. Eggs will continue cooking from residual heat. Let cool slightly and serve with toast, if desired.

Baked French Toast

Ingredients

• 2 tablespoons butter or coconut oil, melted

- 6 eggs

- 1½ cups whole milk

- 2 cups whole-milk ricotta cheese

- 1 tablespoon vanilla extract

- ½ teaspoon salt

- 1 loaf bread, sliced (baguette, white bread, Brioche, or challah)

- ¾ cup apricot or peach preserves, or apple jelly

- ¼ cup heavy cream

- 1 tablespoon powdered sugar (optional)

- Maple syrup

Instructions

- Coat a 9-by-13 baking dish with melted butter.

- In a large bowl, beat eggs, milk, 1 cup ricotta, vanilla, and salt with

a whisk or electric beater.

- Spread each piece of bread with preserves. Arrange bread in two layers, jam-side up, in prepared baking dish. Pour wet ingredients over bread. Cover with plastic wrap or lid and refrigerate overnight.

- Preheat oven to 350 degrees. Bake French toast for 45 minutes for a softer, bread-pudding-like texture or for 1 hour for a firmer, crisper texture. If the top begins browning too quickly, loosely cover with aluminum foil. French toast should register 160 degrees Fahrenheit or higher using an instant-read thermometer placed in the middle of the dish.

- While French toast is baking, whip cream in a large bowl with an electric beater until stiff peaks form. Gently fold in remaining 1 cup ricotta and powdered sugar, if desired.

- Serve French toast warm with whipped ricotta cream and maple syrup.

Banana Pancakes

Ingredients

• 2 large egg whites or ¼ cup liquid egg whites

• 1 ripe medium banana, mashed

• 2 tablespoons instant oats

• ¼ teaspoon cinnamon (optional)

• Cooking spray

• Sugar-free maple syrup, plain yogurt, or creamy nut butter (optional)

Instructions

• In medium bowl, whisk egg whites until frothy. Add banana, oats, and cinnamon, if using, and stir until combined.

• Heat large nonstick skillet over medium heat. Lightly coat pan with cooking spray. Spoon batter onto hot skillet to form three small pancakes. Cook until golden brown, about 2 to 3 minutes per side.

• Add any desired toppings.

Barley Risotto

Ingredients

- 2 tablespoons plus 2 teaspoons olive oil

- 1 shallot, finely minced

- ½ cup dry barley

- 3 cups low-sodium vegetable or chicken stock

- 2 cups peeled and diced butternut squash

- ½ teaspoon salt

- ¼ cup crumbled pasteurized milk feta cheese (optional)

Instructions

- Thoroughly rinse fresh produce under warm running water for 20 seconds. Scrub to remove excess dirt.

• Heat 2 tablespoons olive oil over medium-low heat in a medium saucepan. Add shallot and cook until softened, 3 to 5 minutes. Add barley and stir well to combine so each kernel is coated.

• Increase heat to medium high and toast barley, stirring constantly, for 3 minutes. Add 2 tablespoons stock and stir. Continue to add stock, ¼ cup at a time, while continuing to stir, allowing stock to absorb into barley. Continue adding stock until barley is tender, about 30 minutes.

• While barley is cooking, heat remaining 2 teaspoons olive oil in a small pan. Add butternut squash and salt and cook over low heat until tender and cooked through, about 15 minutes.

• When barley is tender and most of the stock has been absorbed, add cooked butternut squash and stir well to combine. Add feta, if desired.

• To serve, risotto should register 145 degrees Fahrenheit or higher on an instant-read thermometer placed in the middle of the dish.

Refrigerate risotto within one hour of cooking and eat any leftovers within 48 hours.

Black Beans, Corn, and Quinoa Salad

Ingredients

- ½ cup red quinoa

- 1 cup water

- 15-ounce can black beans (1¾ cup cooked)

- 15.25-ounce can corn, drained

- 1 medium red bell pepper, diced

- 1 cup cherry tomatoes, halved

- 2 cloves garlic, minced

- 6 tablespoons extra-virgin olive oil

- 4 tablespoons lime juice

- 1 teaspoon lime zest

• ½ cup fresh cilantro, chopped

• ¼ teaspoon salt

• 1 avocado, diced

Instructions

• Thoroughly rinse fresh produce under warm running water for 20 seconds. Scrub to remove excess dirt.

• Rinse quinoa in a fine-mesh colander under running water for at least 30 seconds. Drain well.

• In a saucepan, bring rinsed quinoa and water to a boil over medium-high heat, then reduce heat and simmer until quinoa has absorbed the liquid, 10 to 12 minutes. Remove pan from heat, cover, and let stand 5 minutes.

• When quinoa is cool, add it to a large bowl with beans, corn, bell pepper, tomatoes, garlic, olive oil, lime juice and zest, cilantro, and salt and mix well. Cover and chill for a few hours or overnight.

• To serve, bring salad to room temperature, add avocado, and mix gently to combine.

Ingredients

• Cooking spray

• 1 small russet potato, peeled and diced

• 8 eggs

• ½ cup cottage cheese

• 2 ounces cheddar cheese, grated

• 1 small bell pepper, chopped

• 2 tablespoons ketchup

Instructions

• Preheat oven to 350 degrees. Grease a 12-cup muffin tin, or line with muffin cups or parchment paper.

• Place potato in a microwave-safe dish, cover, and microwave for 5 minutes. Let sit for 5 minutes.

• In a large mixing bowl, beat eggs. Add cottage cheese, cheddar, bell pepper, ketchup, and cooked potato. Divide mixture evenly into prepared muffin tin.

• Bake until tops are golden, 15 to 18 minutes. Egg cups should register 160 degrees Fahrenheit or higher using an instant-read thermometer placed in the middle of a cup.

Black Beans, Corn, and Quinoa Salad

Ingredients

• ½ cup red quinoa

• 1 cup water

• 15-ounce can black beans (1¾ cup cooked)

• 15.25-ounce can corn, drained

• 1 medium red bell pepper, diced

- 1 cup cherry tomatoes, halved

- 2 cloves garlic, minced

- 6 tablespoons extra-virgin olive oil

- 4 tablespoons lime juice

- 1 teaspoon lime zest

- ½ cup fresh cilantro, chopped

- ¼ teaspoon salt

- 1 avocado, diced

Instructions

- Thoroughly rinse fresh produce under warm running water for 20 seconds. Scrub to remove excess dirt.

- Rinse quinoa in a fine-mesh colander under running water for at least 30 seconds. Drain well.

• In a saucepan, bring rinsed quinoa and water to a boil over medium-high heat, then reduce heat and simmer until quinoa has absorbed the liquid, 10 to 12 minutes. Remove pan from heat, cover, and let stand 5 minutes.

• When quinoa is cool, add it to a large bowl with beans, corn, bell pepper, tomatoes, garlic, olive oil, lime juice and zest, cilantro, and salt and mix well. Cover and chill for a few hours or overnight.

• To serve, bring salad to room temperature, add avocado, and mix gently to combine.

Brown Rice Stir Fry

Ingredients

• ⅓ cup brown rice

• 1 cup water

• 1½ tablespoons olive oil

• 1 3-ounce chicken breast, cut into strips

- 1 cup broccoli florets

- ½ cup onion, sliced

- ½ cup yellow pepper, cut into strips

- ½ cup carrots, cut into strips

Instructions

- Add rice and water to a small pot and bring to a boil over medium-high heat.

- Reduce temperature to medium-low, cover, and simmer until liquid is completely absorbed and rice is tender, about 40 minutes.

- Remove pot from heat and let sit for 10 minutes, then uncover and fluff rice with a fork.

- In a frying pan, heat ¾ tablespoon olive oil.

- Add chicken and heat until cooked or reaches 165 degrees with a meat thermometer.

- Remove chicken from pan and set aside.

- Add remaining oil to pan.

- Add vegetables. Cook for 2 minutes.

- Return chicken to pan and heat for 2 more minutes, or 4 minutes

if you prefer softer vegetables.

- Serve immediately.

Buffalo Cauliflower Bites

Ingredients

- Cooking spray

- 2 medium heads cauliflower, cut into small florets

- 1 cup brown rice flour, chickpea flour, or any flour available

- 1 cup water

- 2 teaspoons garlic powder

- 1 teaspoon salt

- 2 teaspoons butter

- 1 ⅓ cups Frank's Hot Sauce

Instructions

- Thoroughly rinse fresh produce under warm running water for 20 seconds. Scrub to remove excess dirt.

- Preheat oven to 450 degrees. Line a rimmed baking sheet with parchment paper or spray with cooking spray.

- Toss the cauliflower florets with flour, water, garlic powder, and salt. Place on prepared baking sheet and bake 20 minutes.

- In a small saucepan, melt butter with hot sauce. Pour butter mixture over baked cauliflower and toss to coat.

- Return cauliflower to oven and bake another 20 minutes. Internal temperature of cauliflower should be 145 degrees using an instant-read thermometer. Serve warm.

Butternut Squash and Apple Soup

Ingredients

• 2½ cups butternut squash, peeled and cubed

• 4 tablespoons extra-virgin olive oil

• 1 yellow onion, chopped

• 1 clove garlic, minced

• 5 cups low-sodium vegetable stock

• 2 cups water

• 1 16-ounce can pumpkin puree

• 2 medium red apples, peeled and chopped

• ¼ teaspoon ground cinnamon

• ¼ teaspoon ground nutmeg

• ¼ teaspoon ground cloves

• ¼ teaspoon salt

- ½ teaspoon black pepper

- 4 tablespoons low-fat plain Greek yogurt

- Roasted pumpkin seeds (optional)

Instructions

- Thoroughly rinse fresh produce under warm running water for 20 seconds. Scrub to remove excess dirt.

- Preheat oven to 350 degrees.

- Line a rimmed baking sheet with parchment paper, then spread squash evenly on paper. Drizzle squash with 2 tablespoons olive oil and roast 8 to 10 minutes. Remove from oven and set aside.

- Heat remaining 2 tablespoons olive oil in a large pot over medium heat. Add onion and garlic. Cook until onion is soft and starts to brown. Add roasted squash, vegetable stock, water, pumpkin puree, apples, cinnamon, nutmeg, cloves, salt, and black pepper. Bring to a boil over high heat, then reduce to a simmer and cook until squash and apples are tender, about 20 minutes. Remove from heat and let cool.

• Puree soup using an immersion blender, food mill, food processor, or blender. Place pot over low heat until soup is warmed through, about 30 minutes. Add yogurt, stirring until completely combined. Soup should be 145 degrees using an instant-read thermometer.

• Ladle soup into bowls and garnish with seeds, if using.

Cantaloupe and Mint Granita

Ingredients

• 2 cups water

• 1 cup sugar, or more to taste

• 1¼ cup fresh mint leaves

• 1 cantaloupe, peeled, seeded, and chopped

• 3 tablespoons lime juice

Instructions

• Thoroughly rinse fresh produce under warm running water for 20 seconds. Scrub to remove excess dirt.

• In a small saucepan, combine the water, 1 cup sugar, and 1 cup mint leaves. Bring to a boil over medium heat. Reduce heat and simmer, stirring occasionally, until sugar has dissolved, about 5 minutes. Remove pan from heat and set aside to cool, about 20 minutes. Pour cooled syrup through a strainer to remove mint leaves.

• In a blender, puree the strained syrup, cantaloupe, and lime juice until smooth, then taste. To sweeten more, add 1 tablespoon sugar at a time and blend; taste and repeat until desired flavor is reached. Add remaining mint leaves and blend until finely chopped.

• Pour the mixture into a 9x13 glass baking dish and freeze, at least 8 hours or overnight.

• Using the tines of a fork, scrape the granita to the desired texture and serve in chilled bowls.

Butternut Squash and Apple Soup

Ingredients

• 2½ cups butternut squash, peeled and cubed

• 4 tablespoons extra-virgin olive oil

• 1 yellow onion, chopped

• 1 clove garlic, minced

• 5 cups low-sodium vegetable stock

• 2 cups water

• 1 16-ounce can pumpkin puree

• 2 medium red apples, peeled and chopped

• ¼ teaspoon ground cinnamon

• ¼ teaspoon ground nutmeg

- ¼ teaspoon ground cloves

- ¼ teaspoon salt

- ½ teaspoon black pepper

- 4 tablespoons low-fat plain Greek yogurt

- Roasted pumpkin seeds (optional)

Instructions

- Thoroughly rinse fresh produce under warm running water for 20 seconds. Scrub to remove excess dirt.

- Preheat oven to 350 degrees.

- Line a rimmed baking sheet with parchment paper, then spread squash evenly on paper. Drizzle squash with 2 tablespoons olive oil and roast 8 to 10 minutes. Remove from oven and set aside.

- Heat remaining 2 tablespoons olive oil in a large pot over medium heat. Add onion and garlic. Cook until onion is soft and starts to brown. Add roasted squash, vegetable stock, water, pumpkin puree, apples, cinnamon, nutmeg, cloves, salt, and black pepper. Bring to a boil over high heat, then reduce to a simmer and cook until squash and apples are tender, about 20 minutes. Remove from heat and let cool.

• Puree soup using an immersion blender, food mill, food processor, or blender. Place pot over low heat until soup is warmed through, about 30 minutes. Add yogurt, stirring until completely combined. Soup should be 145 degrees using an instant-read thermometer.

• Ladle soup into bowls and garnish with seeds, if using.

Buffalo Cauliflower Bites

Ingredients

• Cooking spray

• 2 medium heads cauliflower, cut into small florets

• 1 cup brown rice flour, chickpea flour, or any flour available

- 1 cup water

- 2 teaspoons garlic powder

- 1 teaspoon salt

- 2 teaspoons butter

- 1 ⅓ cups Frank's Hot Sauce

Instructions

- Thoroughly rinse fresh produce under warm running water for 20 seconds. Scrub to remove excess dirt.

- Preheat oven to 450 degrees. Line a rimmed baking sheet with parchment paper or spray with cooking spray.

- Toss the cauliflower florets with flour, water, garlic powder, and salt. Place on prepared baking sheet and bake 20 minutes.

- In a small saucepan, melt butter with hot sauce. Pour butter mixture over baked cauliflower and toss to coat.

• Return cauliflower to oven and bake another 20 minutes. Internal temperature of cauliflower should be 145 degrees using an instant-read thermometer. Serve warm.

Brown Rice Stir Fry

Ingredients

• ⅓ cup brown rice

• 1 cup water

• 1½ tablespoons olive oil

• 1 3-ounce chicken breast, cut into strips

• 1 cup broccoli florets

• ½ cup onion, sliced

• ½ cup yellow pepper, cut into strips

• ½ cup carrots, cut into strips

Instructions

• Add rice and water to a small pot and bring to a boil over medium-high heat.

• Reduce temperature to medium-low, cover, and simmer until liquid is completely absorbed and rice is tender, about 40 minutes.

• Remove pot from heat and let sit for 10 minutes, then uncover and fluff rice with a fork.

• In a frying pan, heat ¾ tablespoon olive oil.

• Add chicken and heat until cooked or reaches 165 degrees with a meat thermometer.

• Remove chicken from pan and set aside.

• Add remaining oil to pan.

• Add vegetables. Cook for 2 minutes.

• Return chicken to pan and heat for 2 more minutes, or 4 minutes if you prefer softer vegetables.

• Serve immediately.

Ingredients

• Cooking spray

• 2 medium heads cauliflower, cut into small florets

• 1 cup brown rice flour, chickpea flour, or any flour available

• 1 cup water

• 2 teaspoons garlic powder

• 1 teaspoon salt

• 2 teaspoons butter

• 1 ⅓ cups Frank's Hot Sauce

Instructions

• Thoroughly rinse fresh produce under warm running water for 20 seconds. Scrub to remove excess dirt.

• Preheat oven to 450 degrees. Line a rimmed baking sheet with parchment paper or spray with cooking spray.

• Toss the cauliflower florets with flour, water, garlic powder, and salt. Place on prepared baking sheet and bake 20 minutes.

• In a small saucepan, melt butter with hot sauce. Pour butter mixture over baked cauliflower and toss to coat.

• Return cauliflower to oven and bake another 20 minutes. Internal temperature of cauliflower should be 145 degrees using an instant-read thermometer. Serve warm

Butternut Squash and Apple Soup

Ingredients

• 2½ cups butternut squash, peeled and cubed

• 4 tablespoons extra-virgin olive oil

• 1 yellow onion, chopped

• 1 clove garlic, minced

- 5 cups low-sodium vegetable stock

- 2 cups water

- 1 16-ounce can pumpkin puree

- 2 medium red apples, peeled and chopped

- ¼ teaspoon ground cinnamon

- ¼ teaspoon ground nutmeg

- ¼ teaspoon ground cloves

- ¼ teaspoon salt

- ½ teaspoon black pepper

- 4 tablespoons low-fat plain Greek yogurt

- Roasted pumpkin seeds (optional)

Instructions

- Thoroughly rinse fresh produce under warm running water for 20 seconds. Scrub to remove excess dirt.

• Preheat oven to 350 degrees.

• Line a rimmed baking sheet with parchment paper, then spread squash evenly on paper. Drizzle squash with 2 tablespoons olive oil and roast 8 to 10 minutes. Remove from oven and set aside.

• Heat remaining 2 tablespoons olive oil in a large pot over medium heat. Add onion and garlic. Cook until onion is soft and starts to brown. Add roasted squash, vegetable stock, water, pumpkin puree, apples, cinnamon, nutmeg, cloves, salt, and black pepper. Bring to a boil over high heat, then reduce to a simmer and cook until squash and apples are tender, about 20 minutes. Remove from heat and let cool.

• Puree soup using an immersion blender, food mill, food processor, or blender. Place pot over low heat until soup is warmed through, about 30 minutes. Add yogurt, stirring until completely combined. Soup should be 145 degrees using an instant-read thermometer.

• Ladle soup into bowls and garnish with seeds, if using.

Cantaloupe and Mint Granita

Ingredients

• 2 cups water

• 1 cup sugar, or more to taste

• 1¼ cup fresh mint leaves

• 1 cantaloupe, peeled, seeded, and chopped

• 3 tablespoons lime juice

Instructions

• Thoroughly rinse fresh produce under warm running water for 20 seconds. Scrub to remove excess dirt.

• In a small saucepan, combine the water, 1 cup sugar, and 1 cup mint leaves. Bring to a boil over medium heat. Reduce heat and simmer, stirring occasionally, until sugar has dissolved, about 5 minutes. Remove pan from heat and set aside to cool, about 20 minutes. Pour cooled syrup through a strainer to remove mint leaves.

• In a blender, puree the strained syrup, cantaloupe, and lime juice until smooth, then taste. To sweeten more, add 1 tablespoon sugar at a time and blend; taste and repeat until desired flavor is reached. Add remaining mint leaves and blend until finely chopped.

• Pour the mixture into a 9x13 glass baking dish and freeze, at least 8 hours or overnight.

• Using the tines of a fork, scrape the granita to the desired texture and serve in chilled bowls.

Rainbow Grain Bowl with Cashew Tahini Sauce

Ingredients

• ¾ cup unsalted cashews

• ½ cup water

- ¼ cup packed parsley leaves

- 1 tablespoon lemon juice or cider vinegar

- 1 tablespoon extra-virgin olive oil

- ½ teaspoon reduced-sodium tamari or soy sauce (see Tip)

- ¼ teaspoon salt

- ½ cup cooked lentils

- ½ cup cooked quinoa

- ½ cup shredded red cabbage

- ¼ cup grated raw beet

- ¼ cup chopped bell pepper

- ¼ cup grated carrot

- ¼ cup sliced cucumber

- 1 tablespoon Toasted chopped cashews for garnish

Directions

• Blend cashews, water, parsley, lemon juice (or vinegar), oil, tamari (or soy sauce) and salt in a blender until smooth.

• Place lentils and quinoa in the center of a shallow serving bowl. Top with cabbage, beet, pepper, carrot and cucumber. Spoon 2 tablespoons of the cashew sauce over the top (save extra sauce for another use). Garnish with cashews, if desired.

Tips

Tip: People with celiac disease or gluten sensitivity should use soy sauces that are labeled "gluten-free," as soy sauce may contain wheat or other gluten-containing sweeteners and flavors.

Nutrition Facts

Serving Size: 1 bowl

Per Serving: 361 calories; protein 16.6g; carbohydrates 53.9g; dietary fiber 14g; sugars 9g; fat 10.1g; saturated fat 1.7g; vitamin a iu 5999.4IU; vitamin c 68.4mg; folate 291.7mcg; calcium 76.7mg;

iron 6.2mg; magnesium 149.6mg; potassium 941mg; sodium 139.1mg; thiamin 0.4mg.

Herbed Avocado Egg Salad

Replace the mayonnaise with avocado and creamy nonfat Greek yogurt and you have an egg salad that is heart healthy and safe for people following a low-fiber diet. Top on a slide of bread or serve with salad greens.

Prep time 25 minutes

Total Time 25 minutes

Ingredients

- 10 eggs

- 1 avocado

- ½ cup nonfat plain Greek yogurt

- ½ teaspoon Dijon mustard

- Juice of 1 lemon

- 1 tablespoon chopped chives

- 1 tablespoon chopped dill

- Salt and pepper

- 1 tablespoon olive oil

Instructions

- Place eggs in a saucepan and fill with water so eggs are covered. Bring to a boil, then remove from heat and let eggs rest in water for 8 to 10 minutes. Remove eggs from pan and run under cold water. Cool and peel, discarding shells.

- Mash avocado and eggs together until a textured and chunky in consistency. Add yogurt, mustard, lemon juice, and herbs. Season with salt and pepper to taste. Drizzle with olive oil.

- Serve chilled or at room temperature. Transfer salad to a bowl if serving immediately or to an airtight container if saving for later. Store up to three days in the refrigerator.

Lentil soup is always a great option if you're having difficulties swallowing. Fresh rosemary and shallots gives this version its rich, comforting flavor.

Prep time 10 minutes

Cook Time 40 minutes

Total Time 50 minutes

Yield Serves 4

Ingredients

- 2 tablespoons olive oil

- 2 shallots, minced

- 4 large carrots, washed, peeled, and sliced

- 2 cloves garlic, minced

- ½ teaspoon salt

- ½ teaspoon ground black pepper

- 2 sweet potatoes, washed, peeled, and diced

- 4 cups low-sodium vegetable or chicken broth

- 2 to 3 sprigs fresh rosemary, washed well

- 1 cup dry green or brown lentils, thoroughly rinsed and drained

- 2 cups chopped kale, very well washed

Instructions

- Thoroughly rinse fresh produce under warm running water for 20 seconds. Scrub to remove excess dirt.

- Heat a large pot over medium heat. Add olive oil, shallots, and carrots, and cook until carrots begin to soften, about 3 minutes. Add garlic and ¼ teaspoon each salt and pepper. Stir to combine, then cook until vegetables are tender, 4 to 5 minutes. Add sweet potatoes and remaining ¼ teaspoon each salt and pepper. Stir and cook an additional 2 minutes.

• Add broth and rosemary, then increase heat to medium high. Bring to a rolling simmer. Add lentils and stir to combine. Reduce heat to low and simmer, uncovered, until lentils and potatoes are tender, 15 to 20 minutes. Add kale, stir, and cover. Cook an additional 3 to 4 minutes to soften. Taste and adjust flavor by adding salt and pepper as needed.

• To serve, soup should register 145 degrees Fahrenheit or higher using an instant-read thermometer in the middle of the dish.

Mango Lassi

Prep time 10 minutes

Total Time 10 minutes

Yield Serves 2

Ingredients

• 2 cups chopped mango

• ½ cup whole-milk yogurt

- ½ cup coconut milk or whole milk

- 1 teaspoon lime juice

- 1 teaspoon honey

- Pinch of cardamom

- 6 ice cubes

Instructions

- Combine all ingredients in a blender. Pulse until smooth.

Quinoa Salad with Feta

This zesty, versatile dish can be served as a side, appetizer, or even the base of a hearty salad.

Prep time 10 minutes

Cook Time 25 minutes

Total Time 35 minutes

Ingredients

- 2 cups quinoa

- 3½ cups low-sodium chicken or vegetable broth

- 1 cup grape tomatoes, halved

- ⅔ cup chopped fresh parsley

- ½ cup diced cucumber, peeled and seeded

- ½ cup minced red onions

- 4 ounces feta cheese, crumbled

- 3 tablespoons olive oil

- 3 tablespoons red wine vinegar

- 2 cloves garlic, minced

- Juice of 1 lemon

- Salt and pepper

Instructions

• Thoroughly rinse fresh produce under warm running water for 20 seconds. Scrub to remove excess dirt.

• Rinse quinoa in a fine-mesh colander under running water for at least 30 seconds. Drain well.

• In a saucepan, bring rinsed quinoa and broth to a boil. Reduce heat to medium-low, cover, and simmer until quinoa is tender and broth is absorbed, 15 to 20 minutes. Transfer to a large bowl and set aside to cool.

• Add tomatoes, parsley, cucumber, onions, feta, olive oil, vinegar, and garlic to cooled quinoa and mix to combine. Pour lemon juice over quinoa salad and season with salt and pepper to taste. Toss to coat and refrigerate until ready to serve.

Herbed Avocado Egg Salad

Replace the mayonnaise with avocado and creamy nonfat Greek yogurt and you have an egg salad that is heart healthy and safe for people following a low-fiber diet. Top on a slide of bread or serve with salad greens.

Prep time 25 minutes

Total Time 25 minutes

Ingredients

- 10 eggs

- 1 avocado

- ½ cup nonfat plain Greek yogurt

- ½ teaspoon Dijon mustard

- Juice of 1 lemon

- 1 tablespoon chopped chives

- 1 tablespoon chopped dill

- Salt and pepper

- 1 tablespoon olive oil

Instructions

- Place eggs in a saucepan and fill with water so eggs are covered. Bring to a boil, then remove from heat and let eggs rest in water for 8 to 10 minutes. Remove eggs from pan and run under cold water. Cool and peel, discarding shells.

- Mash avocado and eggs together until a textured and chunky in consistency. Add yogurt, mustard, lemon juice, and herbs. Season with salt and pepper to taste. Drizzle with olive oil.

- Serve chilled or at room temperature. Transfer salad to a bowl if serving immediately or to an airtight container if saving for later. Store up to three days in the refrigerator.